DEDICATION

I dedicate this book to all my three angels. You are my ultimate reason why I worked so hard to be where I am today.

TABLE OF CONTENTS

Chapter 1- All Natural Way in Losing Weight

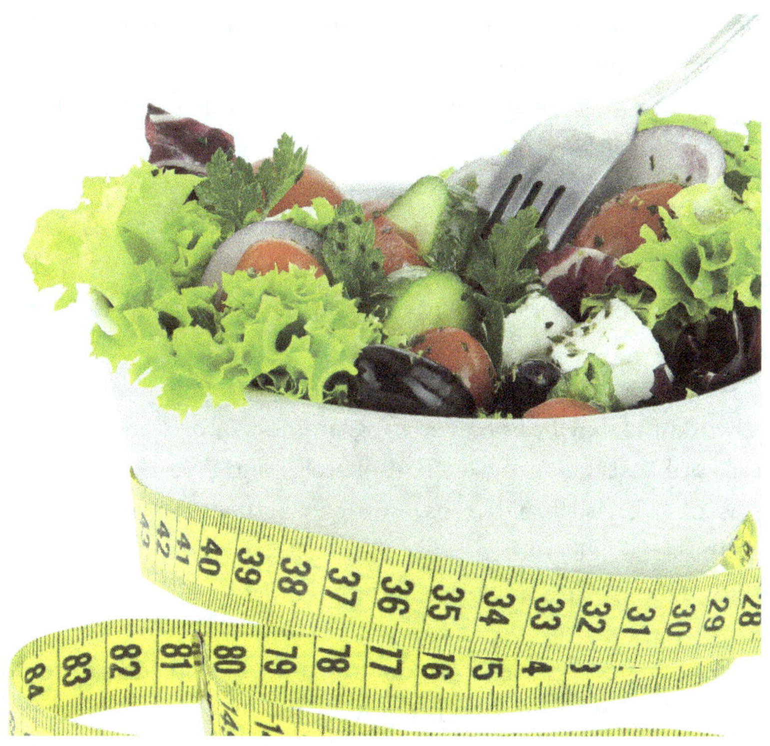

There are no such things as miracle treatments for a weight loss problem. Of course, it is possible to become slim through the use of fad diets, but you will not be healthy because crash diets deny you nutrients that are necessary for your body to function properly.

It weakens your health and what's more you are likely to go back to your former eating habits since the fad diet taught you nothing. You will be having the same problem again and again. Worse, according to studies people who have undergone repetitive weight loss diets, then became permanently overweight, and are in worse health than those who hadn't tried solving their weight problems at all.

Change Your Lifestyle

Changing your lifestyle is actually the most effective way of losing weight and staying healthy. A switch from a calorie-loaded diet to a low calorie diet is a must. You do not actually have to reduce food intake, just eat healthful foods - more vegetables and fruits, lean meats, whole grains and others.

Regular exercise should also help you lose weight as well as maintaining good health. Since you are taking in fewer calories from your diet, your workouts should be burning fat deposits in your body.

The workouts may not be even programmed. Sports and games like tennis or basketball are excellent exercise and if you feel like other forms of exercise are chores. You can actually enjoy the games though, especially when you play with friends, which means turning exercise into a habit will not be difficult.

The process of getting you down to your appropriate weight through the natural method may be slow, but you feel good the whole time and maintaining gains does not require doing anything outside of your established daily routine.

Healthy Eating Habit Tips

In a world where fast food is considered a real meal, no wonder there are so many people in a bad shape. The rate of obese people is a cause for alarm but this can all change if everyone gets educated on healthy eating habits.

The secret to healthy eating is all about balance. It's having all the right nutrients, vitamins and calories in one meal. There's really no need to deprive yourself from food that you like. It's about having

Eat To Lose Weight: Lose Pounds and Beat the Fat Easily

A Guide to Naturally Get the Body that You Want

By: Judy Martin

9781634289801

PUBLISHERS NOTES

Disclaimer – Speedy Publishing LLC

This publication is intended to provide helpful and informative material. It is not intended to diagnose, treat, cure, or prevent any health problem or condition, nor is intended to replace the advice of a physician. No action should be taken solely on the contents of this book. Always consult your physician or qualified health-care professional on any matters regarding your health and before adopting any suggestions in this book or drawing inferences from it.

The author and publisher specifically disclaim all responsibility for any liability, loss or risk, personal or otherwise, which is incurred as a consequence, directly or indirectly, from the use or application of any contents of this book.

Any and all product names referenced within this book are the trademarks of their respective owners. None of these owners have sponsored, authorized, endorsed, or approved this book.

Always read all information provided by the manufacturers' product labels before using their products. The author and publisher are not responsible for claims made by manufacturers.

This book was originally printed before 2014. This is an adapted reprint by Speedy Publishing LLC with newly updated content designed to help readers with much more accurate and timely information and data.

Speedy Publishing LLC

40 E Main Street, Newark, Delaware, 19711

Contact Us: 1-888-248-4521

Website: http://www.speedypublishing.co

REPRINTED Paperback Edition: ISBN: 9781634289801

Manufactured in the United States of America

all of these foods, but in moderation. Like the old saying goes, too much of anything is bad. This can be applied greatly to the food you eat.

The truth is, what you consume everyday greatly affects your whole attitude and energy level for the whole day. Sure it is convenient but there's so much more to life than a cheeseburger meal or Chinese food take out. It's tasty and you can't help craving it, but experimenting in your kitchen can easily result in the best meal of your life.

So here are some tips for healthy eating habits for a better you:

One Step at a Time

If you are just starting to change into a healthier lifestyle, then do it slowly. Your body has been accustomed to old ways and if you change drastically, it is likely that you will also give up easily.

Eat At Home

Whenever you eat out, you do not have any control on the portions that you will have. You might end up eating more than you need to.

Stop Counting the Calories

Do not be obsessed about that. Instead, look at food in terms of color and freshness. Greens are always good. Colorful fruits are also great for a person's body. These are the food that your body needs more of. So do not feel afraid to eat more of these.

Do Not Skip Meals

If your goal is to lose weight, then it is much better to eat small portions of food 5- 6 times a day. Skipping meals will only retain the fat in your body and may result in overeating.

Snack Healthy

When you're feeling hungry, instead of reaching out for the cupcake, grab that carrot stick instead. Some good examples of food to snack on are fruits, nuts, raisins, cranberries, whole grain crackers, etc.

Enjoy Your Meal

Do not rush the eating process. Take your time and chew your food slowly. When you're already feeling full, then stop eating. Listen to what your body tells you.

Remember To Drink a Lot of Water

Sometimes people confuse thirst with hunger and eat when all they needed was just a glass of water. Drinking water is also good for cleansing the body from toxins and helps in having better digestion.

Along with these tips, you should always remember to have not just good eating habits but also a healthy lifestyle. This means making an effort to exercise regularly. If you are a smoker, then consider quitting and lastly, drink alcoholic beverages moderately.

CHAPTER 2- CHOOSE THE RIGHT FOOD TO LOSE WEIGHT

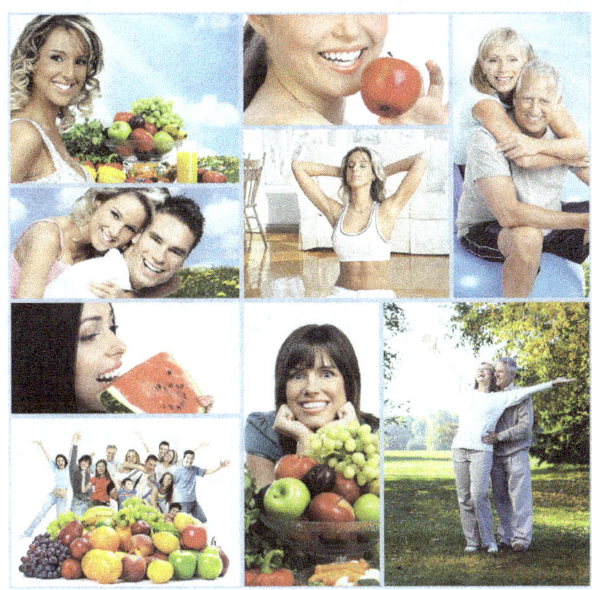

When trying to lose weight, dieters tend to focus on the quantity of the food they intake. If you are one of these people wanting to shed pounds, listen up. Here's something that you need to keep in mind:

CHOOSE QUALITY OVER QUANTITY ALL THE TIME.

Most people on a diet tend to drastically cut down on food. Some even starve themselves thinking if they do not eat food, they won't gain weight. Sure, that is true. However, it will also not help you lose weight. In fact, if you stop eating, your body will work on keeping your fats so that you can have the energy you need during the day.

So what does a person have to do? What is the right quantity of food to eat during a diet? How often can a person eat? All of these questions will be answered in this article, so continue reading on.

Small Portions Several Times throughout the Day

Most experts say that there are many more benefits when it comes to losing weight if you eat 5-6 meals per day compared to 3 meals. Granted the meals are small, of course. The reason for this is because your body will have balanced levels of sugar in the blood. Meaning, you won't be feeling intense hunger. When a person is hungry, they tend to eat more than usual.

Eating smaller portions throughout the day will also reduce cholesterol. In studies done by experts, it was proven that having smaller meals consumed 6 times a day decreased cholesterol levels by 5 percent.

Fill that Plate Up With the Right Kind of Stuff

What a person eats greatly affects their weight loss or weight gain. This is why dietitians encourage people to go for quality over quantity. A good example is you might have eaten only crackers for lunch today but also had a huge jug of sweetened drinks. Then that sweetened drink is the culprit when it comes to your weight gain.

If you had a large bowl of fresh salad and water, then that would have been considered a better meal on a diet than the crackers with a sweetened drink. It is much better for the body to take foods that are less in carbohydrates. Taking away bread, pasta, rice or potatoes and replacing it with vegetables will definitely help cut back on fat.

If you are the type of person who will feel full only if you see large portions of food on your plate, then the solution is to fill your plate with the right kind of food. Think colorful fruits and vegetables. Deep colors means higher content of vitamins, minerals and antioxidants. All of these are what your body needs every day.

To commit to a long-term diet, it is important to like what you eat. If you hate the thought of just eating vegetables or fruits all day, then do some research on diet recipes. Eating meat is encouraged, so don't cut back on that. As long as it is not always deep fried, then it's still good.

It's really important to enjoy the process. Otherwise, you will easily go back to your old routine. Just remember, too much of anything is bad. Keep everything well balanced and eat only when your body is telling you it's hungry.

Have Balanced Diet

If you have noticed, just a quick search of weight loss on the Internet will immediately provide you with weight loss products like diet pills, weight loss programs and even gym memberships. These can cost a great deal of money and most of them are not even effective. So why not go back to basics and do the easiest and the cheapest thing you can do to lose weight: adopt a balanced diet.

Achieving a balanced diet includes eating the right kind and amount of food that will give you enough nutrients to sustain weight loss. Ideally, your diet should be heavier in fruits and vegetables, whole carbohydrates and low in dietary fats.

Additionally, lean proteins, and lots of water for hydration and exercise are important. Even though we all have different nutrient needs and metabolisms, all these factors are still important to achieve weight loss in the safest and cheapest way.

The Benefits of a Balanced Diet

Opting for a balanced diet to maintain a healthy weight is important in order to achieve weight loss since you are still supplying your body the right amount of vitamins and minerals it needs to function properly. When combined with consistent exercise, it is inevitable that you will lose weight without risking any health problems.

Maintaining a balanced diet with the aim of losing weight is beneficial as compared to products that promise a quick and easy way to weight loss. First, it lessens the risk of your developing cardiovascular diseases like heart diseases and diabetes. It can also aid you in controlling these conditions if ever you are suffering from one. This healthy regimen also promotes regular metabolism and a healthy digestive system, which will enable you to lose bad fats and absorb the good ones.

Aside from that, the choice of eating a balanced diet will definitely boost your confidence knowing that you will achieve your desired weight in the healthiest way possible.

How to Start Right

Starting out can be quite a challenge but it should be easy. Always remember the basics of eating more whole-carbohydrates by avoiding foods like chocolates, ice creams, chips, sodas, cookies, cakes and many others. These types of foods contain high amounts of sugar, cholesterol, salt and other unwanted substances.

These foods are also called 'empty calories' since they do not provide nutrients other than calories. Choose to drink fresh fruit juice instead of sodas, as they add approximately 500 calories more to your diet.

With that in mind, plan your meal correctly by adding more of the good kinds of food. You can have a high-fiber cereal with low-fat milk at breakfast, and then lunch would be a grilled turkey sandwich over whole wheat bread and a vegetable salad. Dinner can be baked fish and vegetables.

These are just a few of the simple dishes you can make and they are even easier to prepare. Just keep in mind that every meal should contain a variety of foods, such as fruits, lean proteins, vegetables and high-fiber carbohydrates.

CHAPTER 3- WEIGHT LOSS AND BLOOD TYPE PRINCIPLE

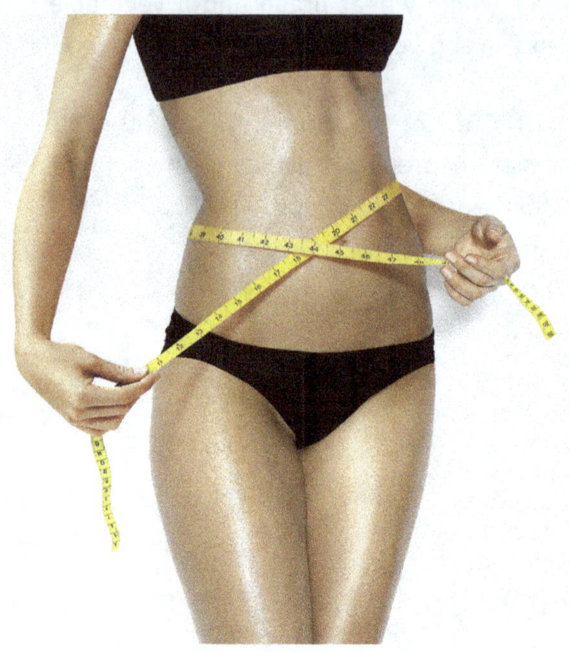

A lot of people now understand the importance of having a healthy body. This is why there is a surge in the health and fitness industry. A lot more people are now going to the gym to try different forms of exercise to get in shape.

People are also trying different kinds of diets, from Atkins to Paleo to South Beach to Weight Watchers. All of these are effective, though some more than others. But did you know that there's a diet that is designed for your blood type? If you have tried almost all of the famous diet trends available and have not seen a lot of results, then this might be the perfect one for you.

This diet was designed by Doctor Peter D'Amado and is called The Blood Group Diet. This new diet is gaining more popularity because a lot of the big names in Hollywood say it's the reason for their amazing bodies. Actors like Courtney Cox and Cheryl Cole swear by it.

So what exactly is The Blood Group Diet and how does it work?

It is believed that each blood group reacts differently to each food. So if you follow the diet designed for you, the chances of losing weight will be higher because your body will absorb food more efficiently.

Let's look at the diet closely. If you have Blood Type O, which is the most common blood type in humans, then the diet should be similar to Paleo where it is encouraged to eat more like "hunter-gatherer" style. This means eating food that was available to our ancestors before agriculture growth and advancement in technology happened. High protein and low in carbohydrates is the way to go.

Along with this diet, blood type O people should also do a lot of high intensity cardio like running to complement the diet.

Blood Type a diet is almost the opposite of the diet suggested to Blood Type O. Meaning, their bodies are much more accepting to the more "modern" food. A vegan diet is encouraged, so this means lots of vegetables and carbohydrates like rice, pasta and cereals. However, meat and dairy products such as milk, cheese or butter should be avoided. Meat should be taken in very little quantity.

Blood type a diet is best done with slow and relaxing exercise such as yoga or Pilates.

Blood Type AB can be defined as the most lenient diet. This rare blood type works well with almost every food but with moderation.

Eat to Lose Weight

They have a good immune system, which means they can handle dairy, meat and carbs well. However, vegetables are the most encouraged food to eat. The rest should be eaten in little portions.

When it comes to exercises, Blood type AB should combine both calming and high intensity workouts.

Blood Type B has the least restrictions. Vegetables, fruits, meat, dairy, seafood, and rice - these can all be taken as long as it's part of a balanced diet and not taken in big quantities. The only food to avoid is processed foods such as the ones that can be bought in a can (luncheon meat, hotdog, ham etc)

Any activity that involves exercising the brain such as tennis, golf, and hiking is the best form of exercise for this blood type.

What Science has to Say on Weight Loss

Weight loss can sometimes be tiring. After thousands of dollars spent on diet programs with all efforts to cut-down calories, it seems that you are not losing weight as you expect it.

Of course, you will then have to check with your doctor or nutritionist to see why you are not losing that much weight and you will end up with 'the look' that strikes the paranoia out of you.

These are just few of the challenges you may encounter when you are into weight loss programs. It can get the best out of you depending on how you take all the challenges up. Well, there is a better way to actually achieve weight loss with 3 easy reminders.

The Science

1. There Is Such a Thing Called 'Real Carbohydrates'

The first thing you need to do is to identify your carbohydrate intake. All of us know that carbohydrates are the main source of energy as carbs are readily converted to glucose, the main substance that is used for energy production. All the excess carbohydrates are turned into fat when they aren't used as energy. Now, what you need to remember is that you need to consume 'real carbohydrates' by choosing foods that are not processed. Replace the processed carbohydrates with natural ones like vegetables and fruits in every meal. Momentarily avoid other carbohydrates like chips, breads, pasta, fast food meals and others.

2. Have you ever heard of high-biological proteins? Choose them among others.

High-biological proteins are what you can think of as complete proteins. They are called such because they contain complete amino acids to provide efficient functions in terms of repairing body tissues and supplying proteins to every muscle in your body. Amino acids work like a team: when one is missing, they cannot function well. So it is good to invest in high-biological proteins by eating natural and grass-fed meats and produce. This includes turkey, beef, chicken, lamb, pork and other animal proteins.

3. There are healthy fats, of course.

If you think that fats are the only culprits of weight gain, you are definitely wrong. Your body also needs fats in order to function well as these substances contribute to temperature control, metabolism regulation and lubrication of vein and arteries. So, have a moderate intake of healthy fats, including avocadoes, coconut oil, olive oil, nuts, olives, seeds and butter. Just remember to consume about 2-3 teaspoons of these fats at every meal.

These are the three easy steps that you can always remember for you to have a significant weight loss. Start on these rules and you are off to a good start. It is good to remember that metabolism is as complex as our brain, so the notion of calorie counting does not really apply to all.

The basis of a healthy weight should come from consuming the right amount and kinds of food or to simply put it: the right balance of food. So start your meal right today by investing more on real carbohydrates, high-biological proteins and healthy fats.

Effects of Protein to Weight Loss

When you have just trained so intensely, especially after resting for a while, then you are more prone to get sore muscles a day after your training. Muscle soreness can be very burdensome, as you experience pain in every move you make. With that, you should know all the reasons behind sore muscles and what you can do to prevent them. Well, the basis of this is the consumption of proteins.

The Essence of Protein on Muscles

Proteins are essential to help tissues repair themselves and supply a leaner body structure. There are so many uses of proteins you may never know. In fact, they can also be used as energy when the carbohydrate sources are empty. Aside from that, they strengthen your immune system and give you skin that is smooth in texture. It has anti-aging benefits, enhances memory and so much more. This is why proteins are pretty valuable and should be saved for their functions instead of using them as energy.

The Right Kind of Proteins

Choosing the right kind of protein is essential to give you the advantage of having a lean body mass without the risk of sore muscles. The advice below is from an expert trainer, Taoist master Tommy Kirchhoff. He studied the popular martial arts Sheng Long Fu and is the Grandmaster of Victor Sheng Long Fu. He is a versatile fitness expert and is credited for contributing effective advice to fitness enthusiasts.

Not all have known this fact: proteins are made to function equally as compared to carbohydrates and fats.

So people are so wrong when they just invest in eating chicken alone. All proteins are a definite cure for intense training and they should be eaten in the most absorbable form.

Why?

This is because muscles need an immediate source of protein to supply their needs, especially during a heavy workout. With that, you need to opt for protein powders, as they give the quickest and most absorbable type of proteins to work and repair your body tissues. In order to find out which powdered proteins are best for you, just visit your personal trainer or sports nutritionist. You can also visit a sports house in your area or GNC stores.

Now, if you don't just have the right budget to buy these powdered proteins, which can be expensive by the way, you can opt for egg whites. The only thing that you should remember is this: you have to eat them raw and fresh.

Yes, you can get the most amino acids in raw fresh eggs as compared to cooking them. The reason for this is because as soon as you cook the egg, the structure of its proteins changes significantly, making it less absorbable. So manipulating an egg white, even if you shake, blend or stir them has effects that you may never know. In fact, your body may not even use the proteins completely.

Therefore, whenever you need the best proteins next to the powdered ones, get fresh eggs, separate the yolks (since they contain too much fat and cholesterol) and swallow them up.

Chapter 4 - Importance of Eating On Time

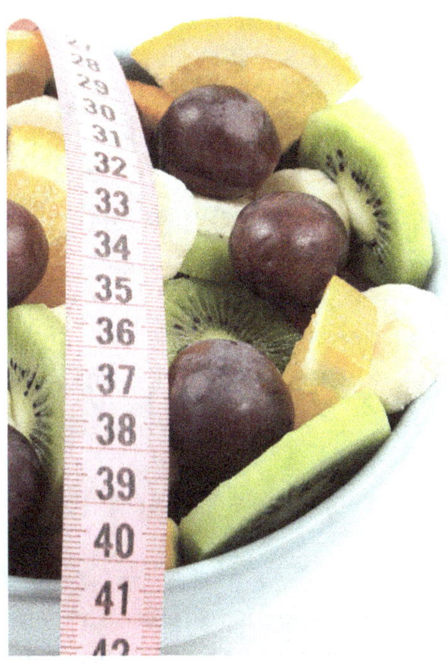

Meal timing is an essential part of a balanced diet. When we want to be on the top of our shapely figure, the right kind, amount and timing is important to balance your calories throughout the day. With that, there is no need to restrict yourself from eating lesser foods or depriving your body with the needed ingredients it should use for a day's work.

Our metabolism is different like our identity. Every individual has a different health and lifestyle profile which explains why it is hard to follow a single diet program.

A diet plan may be effective for you, but not for your friend. Even the intensity and duration of exercise may not be suitable for your friend as compared to yours. So to better understand what is actually happening inside your body, here is a basic explanation.

Timing

Breakfast Time:

The body has fasted from sleep so there is no food intake for 8-12 hours.

With this occurrence, the energy reserves (in the form of glycogen) are definitely low.

This is where our muscles are in a state called mild catabolic, since the energy reserves are used for energy while there is no food intake for 8-12 hours.

The fat stores are being used up as energy. Thus, it is being burned and mobilized.

Your metabolic goal at this time is to replenish the glycogen stores that were used from the fasting hours. You also need to stop your muscles from catabolism so that you will not acquire a state of muscle wasting. Along with that, you also need to support the continuous metabolism of fat.

To do that, you need to have a combination of high quality proteins that are absorbable enough to quickly replenish your muscles from fasting, like eggs and lean meats. You can also mix simple with complex carbohydrates to quickly replenish energy and at the same time, gradually release some of it as you go along your daily routine.

Fat is also important, so make sure to consume essential fatty acids. With that, you can eat walnuts, seeds and avocadoes. You can also make use of little amount of oil like canola oil or flax seed oil.

AM Snack

The level of your glucose is already gradually balancing out

The feeling of hunger is increased

Your metabolic goal: give your muscles the strength they need by consuming proteins and enough carbohydrates. It is good to further balance out your glucose level and at the same time, replenishes protein stores.

To do that: You need to mix proteins and carbohydrates just enough to attain your metabolic goal. Consider foods with low-glycemic index and you can drink protein shakes, whey proteins from milk and fresh egg whites.

Lunch Time

The morning snack that you have eaten is burned as energy and you may need more for a full day's work.

Your metabolic goal is to provide your muscles with sufficient calories with carbohydrates and proteins. Lunch can be your largest meal as compared to breakfast and dinner since you will work more after.

To do this, simply mix high-protein meat products like beef or chicken, then opt for high-fiber and low-glycemic carbohydrates. It is also good to invest in essential fatty acids.

PM Snack

The levels of the glucose in your body are now deteriorating.

With a few hours of mild fasting, your muscle is in a metabolic state again.

At this time, your metabolic goal is to gradually level your glucose up and stop the muscles from being catabolized.

To do this: Simply choose a snack that is enough to keep you replenished until dinner. Eat proteins that are slowly absorbed like cooked eggs. As for the carbohydrates, choose the ones that are low in sugar but are dense in calories.

Dinner Time

Your muscles are anabolic as they prepare for another 8-12 hours of fasting during a sleep. This is up until about 12 in the morning.

Your metabolic goals should support your muscles while they are in an anabolic stage so the catabolic state will not impose any health problems in the long run.

With that, you need to eat types of foods that are low in calories but rich in protein. Choose proteins that are slowly absorbed like beef, pork and chicken. Invest in high-fiber carbohydrates and essential fatty acids.

Stop Counting Calories

Right now, if reports from health agencies are accurate, there could be a billion people in the planet experiencing weight problems. The health and fitness industry which generates billions of dollars in health related revenues continues to churn out various weight loss programs based on drastically reduced calorie diets along with strenuous workouts, and you wonder why the obesity rates are still increasing and whether such an approach is really effective.

Many of the makers of these programs, of course, stress that in order for them to work you heed to persevere, be disciplined and have the tenacity to persist in the face of difficulties that said programs are liable to bring in.

Perhaps the difficulties that you have to undergo when employing these weight loss routines is the main problem which means that all along makers may have been selling an approach that hardly works in the first place. Lose weight fast? You or anyone else for that matter will have a hard time resisting that kind of marketing pitch.

Calorie Deficit, a New and More Effective Approach

Fortunately, some weight loss advocates are trying to shift approaches, from low-calorie diets to less stressful methods. And they base the shift on something that's simple and logical – calorie deficit.

When you are overweight, it only means one thing; you have fat deposits in your body that your metabolism can't process. The question is why your metabolism can't do that. The answer is you are taking more calories than your metabolism can handle. Does this mean that you have to starve yourself in order to lose weight? Of course not, you will be risking your health if you do that and you will end up dealing with worse problems than before.

Eat to Lose Weight

The key to losing weight without experiencing a whole range of issues is to create a calorie deficit, which simply means that you eat fewer calories than your body demands. Fewer calories are the keywords, not zero-calories. When you take in fewer calories and you work out, your body starts burning your fat deposits to supply you with the energy you need for the workouts. Naturally when your body burns fat deposits every day you will not be far away from your ideal weight.

Advantages

The calorie deficit approach has many advantages that are not present in drastically reduced weight loss diets. You do not need specially prepared meals to ensure the required calorie intake levels. All you need to is to eliminate some of the calorie loaded foods you are in the habit of eating. Your body won't be deprived of energy which allows it to function normally and you will feel good as you lose weight.

Aside from reducing the calories, your diet has to be as nutritionally balanced as you can make it. You want the natural body cleansers in it to help your metabolism work more efficiently. You need the proteins and other nutrients that promote good health.

Benefits

One of the benefits of the calorie deficit approach to losing weight is your health is never compromised; instead, you can become healthier. And unlike low calorie diets that make it difficult for you to protect gains because the deprivation will make the foods you used to eat hard to resist, with this approach since its slower the diet will be a habit by the time you have realized your weight reduction goals.

Chapter 5- Are You Obese or Overweight?

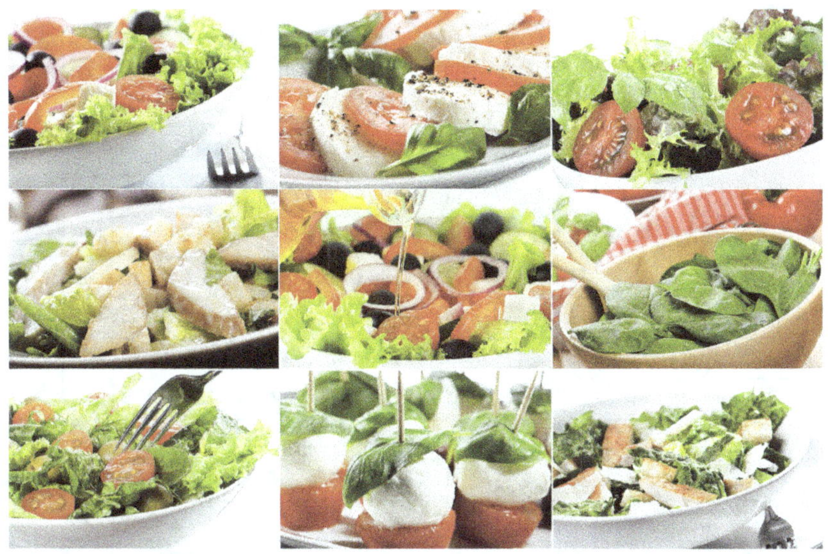

When someone is overweight, their weight exceeds the normal standards for people of their height and age. However, because everyone's weight must include their bones, muscles, fat and water content, it is possible for someone to be overweight without being obese.

For example, a professional athlete or bodybuilder may well be overweight, but because the majority of the 'excess' weight that they are carrying is muscle tissue, they are not obese.

Nevertheless, in the majority of cases, being overweight does equate to carrying too much body fat and often progresses to become clinical obesity.

There are several ways of defining obesity, but the most common is by reference to what is known as 'Body Mass Index' (BMI) which is a mathematical formula that generates a numerical BMI based on

Eat to Lose Weight

an individual's weight in kilograms divided by their height in meters squared. Hence, the mathematical formula for BMI is kg/m2.

BMI (kg/m^2)	19	20	21	22	23	24	25	26	27	28	29	30	35	40
Height (in.)	Weight (lb.)													
58	91	96	100	105	110	115	119	124	129	134	138	143	167	191
59	94	99	104	109	114	119	124	128	133	138	143	148	173	198
60	97	102	107	112	118	123	128	133	138	143	148	153	179	204
61	100	106	111	116	122	127	132	137	143	148	153	158	185	211
62	104	109	115	120	126	131	136	142	147	153	158	164	191	218
63	107	113	118	124	130	135	141	146	152	158	163	169	197	225
64	110	116	122	128	134	140	145	151	157	163	169	174	204	232
65	114	120	126	132	138	144	150	156	162	168	174	180	210	240
66	118	124	130	136	142	148	155	161	167	173	179	186	216	247
67	121	127	134	140	146	153	159	166	172	178	185	191	223	255
68	125	131	138	144	151	158	164	171	177	184	190	197	230	262
69	128	135	142	149	155	162	169	176	182	189	196	203	236	270
70	132	139	146	153	160	167	174	181	188	195	202	207	243	278
71	136	143	150	157	165	172	179	186	193	200	208	215	250	286
72	140	147	154	162	169	177	184	191	199	206	213	221	258	294
73	144	151	159	166	174	182	189	197	204	212	219	227	265	302
74	148	155	163	171	179	186	194	202	210	218	225	233	272	311
75	152	160	168	176	184	192	200	208	216	224	232	240	279	319
76	156	164	172	180	189	197	205	213	221	230	238	246	287	328

So, now you have a BMI figure, what does it mean? From the same web site, you can see the relationship between your clinical weight classification and the risk of weight related illnesses and disease:

Risk of Associated Disease According to BMI and Waist Size			
BMI		Waist less than or equal to 40 in. (men) or 35 in. (women)	Waist greater than 40 in. (men) or 35 in. (women)
18.5 or less	Underweight	--	N/A
18.5 - 24.9	Normal	--	N/A
25.0 - 29.9	Overweight	Increased	High
30.0 - 34.9	Obese	High	Very High
35.0 - 39.9	Obese	Very High	Very High
40 or greater	Extremely Obese	Extremely High	Extremely High

The most common way of quantifying whether someone is obese or not is if their BMI is in excess of 30 points on these scales.

What is Losing Weight Nature's Way all about?

It is no big secret that after 'make money online' information, the #1 category of information that people are searching for on the internet is weight loss related information.

Consequently, it is also no surprise that there are millions of dollars being spent every day on advertising all sorts of diet plans (of widely varying credibility and effectiveness), weight loss wonder pills and equipment - all of which is supposed to help you lose weight - such as exercise machines, multi-gyms etc.

Some of the diet plans that are advertised are entirely natural but the majorities are not. Similarly, most diet pills are not formulated using only natural substances.

Eat to Lose Weight

There is no shortage of businesses that are advertising their weight loss surgery services, many of them in overseas countries where the cost of medical treatment and attention is considerably less than it is in most Western countries.

While you will read of some almost 'too-good-to-be-true' weight loss surgery success stories, you are far less likely to hear anything about the hundreds of cases where weight loss surgery was ultimately ineffective. It is also a fact that undergoing surgery when you are seriously overweight or obese carries significantly heightened risks, but this again is something that you don't hear about.

Taking chemical-based diet pills or undergoing invasive and thoroughly unpleasant surgery is not natural in any way.

So, now you have a fairly clear idea of some weight loss strategies that could in no way qualify as being natural, let's start to look at the flipside.

Natural weight loss Natural weight loss Natural weight loss Natural weight loss Natural weight loss Natural weight loss Natural weight loss Natural weight loss Natural weight loss Natural weight loss Natural weight loss Natural weight loss is a really is a really is a really is a really is a really is a really is a really simple simple simple concept... concept... concept...

The concept that underpins weight loss or indeed weight gain is a very simple one.

Every human being at every stage of their life needs to take in a certain amount of energy in order to get through the day. This energy comes from the nutrition that we take in, in the form of the food we eat or the liquids we drink, and is generally measured in terms of calories or kilocalories. There is a slight difference between the specific meanings accorded to these two terms, with the latter being favored by professional nutritionists, but for the purposes of this book, I am going to use calories as an all-encompassing unit of food energy.

While every individual is different, you need a certain amount of food energy calories every day to satisfy your own personal energy requirements. These requirements will vary according to the amount of physical work you do, how much exercise you take, the speed at which your body burns the energy you are taking on board (your metabolic rate) and your general lifestyle.

However, at the end of the day, if you take on board the right amount of calories every day, your weight will stay stable and you will in general remain healthy.

If you take in too much energy, you will put weight on, but if you take in too little, you will see the opposite effect and lose weight.

It really is as straightforward as this.

You will see diet plans that recommend that you must cut down on your carbohydrates in order to lose weight, with other diet 'experts' on the opposite side of the fence who swear that the only way to lose weight is to reduce the amount of fats in your diet.

However, no matter what type of food you are eating for energy (which includes both carbohydrates and fats), you are going to keep getting fatter as long as you are taking in more energy than you burning. Thus, you will only lose weight if you are taking in less energy than you need.

Eat to Lose Weight

That really is it. That is how you lose weight naturally – you ingest less energy than you need every day, and the fat will gradually fall off.

How much energy do you need? How much energy do you need? How much energy do you need? How much energy do you need? How much energy do you need? How much energy do you need? How much energy do you need? How much energy do you need? How much energy do you need? How much energy do you need? How much energy do you need? How much energy do you need? How much energy do you need? How much energy do you need?

Everyone is different. In addition to our physical attributes, every individual has different energy requirements. In addition, there is some evidence that ability to lose or gain weight is to some extent predetermined by your genetic makeup, and there is not a great deal that you can do about changing that.

On top of your genes, there are many external factors that affect how many calories you need, so any standardized 'calorie table' can be nothing other than a very general, broad brush indication of the number of calories that you need. However, the following are generally accepted to be 'starting point' guidelines:

Sex	Activity Level	Calories Required
	Sedentary	2400
Male	Moderate	2800
	Heavy	3800
	Sedentary	1900
Female	Moderate	2100
	Heavy	3000

In order to get a more accurate picture of exactly how many calories you need, you need to factor in many variables, and after considering what these variables are, you will see how you do this.

Firstly, there are the lifestyle factors to take into account, such as the work that you do, the exercise you take and so on.

These are to a large extent taken into account in the underlying calculation on which the previous chart is based. Someone who is working in a sedentary office based occupation is going to need considerably fewer calories every day than someone who is working on a building site, as an example.

In addition to this, however, your present weight and age will also have an influence on the number of calories you need to maintain your current weight levels.

The more weight you are carrying, the more energy you need to get that bulk moving, while as you get older, your energy requirements gradually decrease as you are likely to engage in less physically activity than you did when you were younger.

Gender is also an influential factor, because women generally need fewer calories than men.

Taking all of these variables into account, what you are looking to do is calculate a 'Body Mass Ratio' (BMR) which is not the same as the 'Body Mass Index' that we were considering earlier.

What BMR does is provide an alternative method for calculating your daily calorific requirements taking account of variables like age, gender, occupation and present weight.

Chapter 6- The Perfect Timing to Losing Weight Naturally

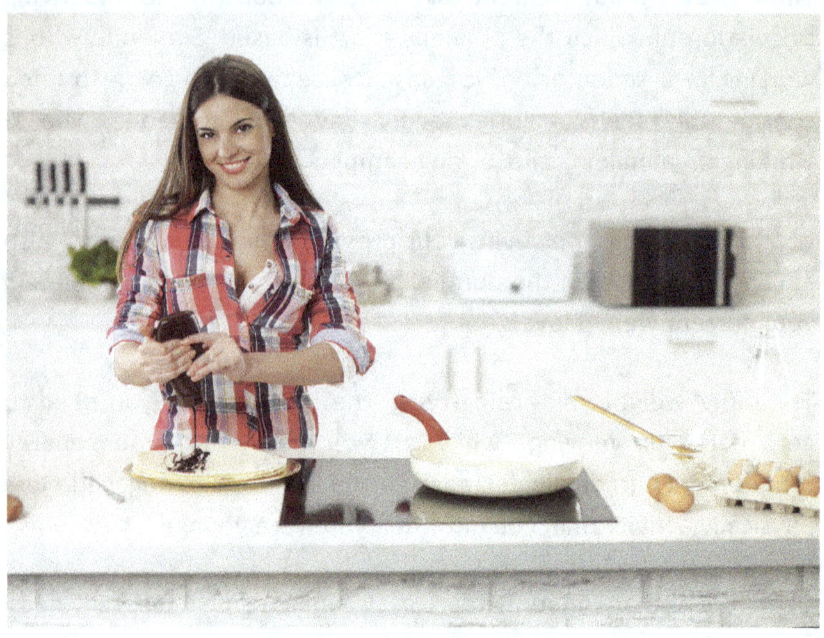

Part of our natural, basic human makeup means that we tend to store fat. In fact, this is something that has been with us for many thousands of years as it was probably a survival mechanism to get over the times when our ancient forebears were short of food.

Given that it is only in recent times that food has become so abundantly plentiful (at least for those of us who live in the West), we have never really lost the capacity for storing unused energy as body fat.

It is a little like animals that hibernate for the winter. They build up a huge store of unused energy during the summer that is sufficient to keep their inactive body 'ticking over' during the winter months when they are hibernating.

You cannot change, nor can you ignore, thousands of years of evolution. The fact is, modern Western man (and woman) has no real need to store unused energy in the way that our prehistoric forebears did, but you are going to continue doing so despite this.

So, if you are taking on too much energy, you are going to get fat, there is no avoiding this. You therefore need to know an awful lot more about why it happens if you want to tackle your problem entirely naturally.

The first thing that you need to understand about losing weight is that almost everything you eat and drink contains calories. The only exception to this rule in terms of naturally occurring substances is water (more about water later).

Other than that, everything you consume contains calories, and it doesn't really matter a great deal how these calories are taken. This is one of the reasons why there are so many virulent arguments between those who suggest that in order to lose weight, you need to cut down on carbohydrates and those who on the other hand suggest that fats are the real demon that needs to be banished from your diet, and why they are probably on the wrong track.

There is little quantifiable scientific proof that following one particular eating approach like this is likely to be more effective for losing weight than anything else. While it is not at all difficult to find seemingly qualified people like medical doctors who will tell you that one particular diet regime (e.g. a carbohydrate only diet) is going to help you lose weight more quickly than anything else, it is surely no coincidence that most of these 'objective' observers have some kind of vested interest in the product or proposal that they are supporting.

Eat to Lose Weight
The fact is, both carbohydrates and fats are processed by the body to produce energy, and so it follows that if you eat too many of either one or the other or even both, you are going to put more weight on.

It does not matter a great deal what kind of foodstuffs or drinks are being taken in to accumulate these extra pounds or kilos - for every excess pound of weight you are dragging around, you must take in 3500 calories less than you need to drop that pound.

However, there is one other thing to take into account, which does lend some credence to the people who suggest that taking in energy in 'form A' (e.g. fats) rather than in 'form B' (e.g. carbohydrates) makes you less fat.

This is the fact that our bodies have the ability to process some calories in one way while dealing with others in a completely different manner.

For example, almost despite what we are generally led to believe, our bodies do not necessarily extract all the goodness (vitamins, nutrients etc) or all of the calories from every single item of food we consume.

This happens because your body has its own metabolic rate, a speed at which it processes the food that you take in.

At the same time, while any foodstuff is still within your body, your body will keep extracting as many calories of energy from that food as possible. Consequently, it follows that anyone whose system passes the food through very quickly is going to draw less calories from their food than would someone whose system is more lethargic.

It is probably no great secret that the modern Western diet is far too rich in processed, refined foods and far too light on raw, nutrient packed foodstuffs. We probably all understand that processed foods (burgers, hot dogs, pizzas etc) are likely to make you fatter than raw unprocessed foods, but one of the reasons why this happens is probably not widely understood.

Partially because these foodstuffs are very rich in fats and sugar, our system is simply not very good at processing them. Consequently, they can hang around in your body for two or three days, and while they are still being slowly digested in this way, your body is still leeching every available calorie from them.

Raw foodstuffs on the other hand tend to 'hang around' for only a few hours and therefore, even if they were 'calorie rich' (which most raw foods are not), your body simply does not get the chance to extract those calories.

When you think about it in these terms, it probably makes a great deal of sense. After all, you have spent years listening to people who have told you how good raw and unprocessed foods were for your digestive system. Plus, there have probably been times when the speed at which you have had to visit the bathroom has provided ample testament to the fact that raw food 'keep you going'!

Now you understand why, and you can probably understand why processed or refined foods are likely to help pile the weight on as well. You'll learn more about this concept later.

In contrast, there are other foodstuffs like the essential fatty acids (the Omega-3 and Omega-6 families) that are never likely to add a great deal of fat to your frame no matter how much of them you eat because their primary function is to help with the repair of bodily cells as well as helping to keep many essential metabolic processes functioning correctly.

So, refined foods are likely to add more weight than are natural raw foods even if they have no difference in terms of total calorific value.

You now know what you have to do to start shifting your unwanted flesh – you have to drop around 3500 calories to get rid of one pound of weight or 7700 calories for every kilo.

Here is a final thing to consider before moving on, one very important thing that you must do before embarking on your fat loss program.

It is extremely important that when you initially start your weight loss regime – hopefully immediately after reading this book – you have a final target weight as an objective.

If you do not have a final objective in mind when you start, it is going to be almost impossible for you to ever feel satisfied with the weight that you have lost and the shape you are in.

It can be extremely tempting to just keep losing weight for the sake of it and that is not the way to good health, fitness and general well-being. On the contrary, it is the way to acquiring anorexia, and while I have no doubt that anyone who is seriously overweight or obese might like to believe that they would welcome being anorexic, it is definitely not something you should want.

Without a final target weight in mind, it is far too easy to become obsessed with losing just a pound or two more until one day someone points out to you that you are already way too thin, by which time it is likely that anorexia is already a problem.

I know that you are probably reading these words thinking 'that could never happen to me' but that are what every anorexic person thinks.

So, taking account of your build, bone structure and musculature, try to establish a 'good weight' (note, not an 'ideal' weight – it does not exist) for someone of your build using a weight table such as this or a downloadable, printable chart like this one, and make that your target.

Having done so, stick to that target so that once you get there, you alter your weight loss diet and exercise regime to one that is designed to maintain weight rather than lose it.

Okay, with that note of caution out of the way, let's start to consider what you can do to get rid of those extra pounds.

The answer is really simple... You pile on the poundage because you are taking in energy that you are not using.

There are two things that you can do to start shedding the fat pounds, two things that can be done in isolation but which work far better if done together.

One is to increase the amount of calories that you burn every day through a program of sensible exercise.

The second is to reduce the calories that you take in, so that instead of eating more calories than you need every day, you are eating fewer.

As suggested, these could be considered an 'either/or' choice, but I would strongly suggest that you should think about both at the same time, because doing so cannot fail to accelerate the speed at which you will shed the extra pounds.

We will begin by looking at the benefits of exercise.

Chapter 7- Sweat it Out and Lose Weight Fast

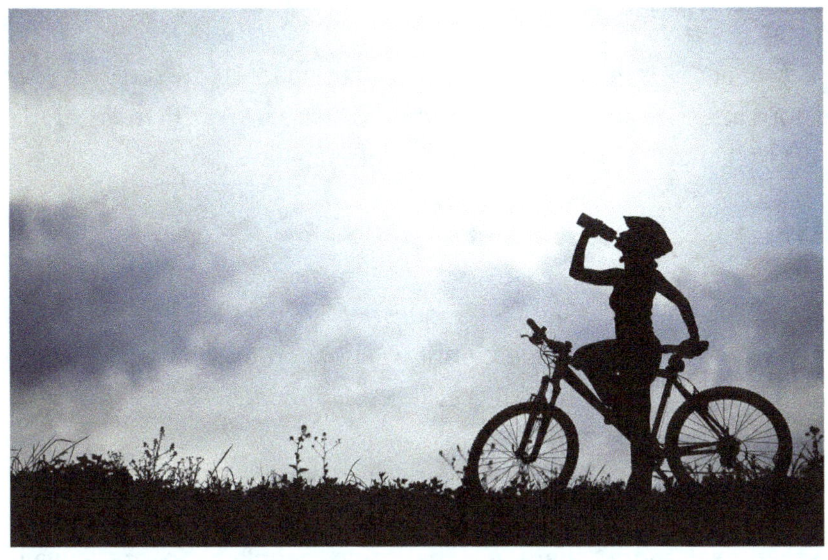

Why exercise helps weight loss in more ways than one

The benefit of exercise is that while you are exercising, you will be burning additional calories over and above those that you have been using previously.

Consequently, exercise will help to get rid of the additional weight you are carrying. If regular exercise and you have become strangers in the recent past, it is time to start getting yourself reacquainted with doing some exercise.

However, it goes much further than actually burning off more calories when you are participating in exercise, because activity helps to speed up your metabolism as well.

In essence, once you start a program of regular exercise, your body might actually burn more calories even when at rest, so that there will be an all-round improvement in the speed at which you are using up the calories. In fact, this improvement can go as far as burning off more calories when you sleep, because although your body is at rest, the 'speed up' effect in your metabolism is a 24/7 thing.

However, it is generally believed that anaerobic exercise is far more effective for burning fat when you are at rest than is aerobic exercise. I will expand on the differences below.

What kind of exercise is best?

There is no one answer to the question of what kind of exercise is best, because to a large extent it will depend on what you want to achieve while getting rid of the surplus poundage.

For example, while most overweight people are likely to be primarily interested in getting rid of their surplus fat and not a great deal more, there will be some people who are equally interested in building their musculature.

For anyone that falls into this category, the exercises that you choose to do will be different from those that work best for people who are just trying to shed the extra pounds of fat. As an example, if you are trying to replace fat with muscle, then lifting weights is going to be more appropriate than would be swimming or running, although of course, all three forms of exercise would have significant benefits.

In essence therefore, you need to know what your primary target is before deciding what kind of exercise program is best for you.

There are essentially two different types of exercise, aerobic and anaerobic.

Aerobic exercise is called this because it encompasses the exercises that make you 'out of breath', so that you begin breathing more deeply as a way of replacing the depleted levels of oxygen in your body and blood. Aerobic exercise works your lungs and speeds up your heart, and it is therefore generally better at burning fat than is anaerobic exercise. Aerobic exercise takes in such things as running or jogging, swimming, cycling and even walking.

Anaerobic exercise on the other hand is the opposite, the kind of exercise that does not get you out of breath or makes you 'puff and pant'. Falling into this category would be the weightlifting. As previously suggested, anaerobic exercise does not burn off the fat as quickly as does aerobic, but it does have the benefit that it is more effective for speeding up your metabolism, leading to the effect of burning more calories even when at rest.

Aerobic exercise works as part of a fat burning weight loss plan, because your body normally turns to carbohydrates to provide the energy that you need. However, when exercising, your body starts to look to the stored fat to provide some of the necessary energy as well, hence the weight loss effect.

Anaerobic exercise on the other hand will generally be almost entirely fuelled by the carbohydrates in your body, and therefore the fat loss effect is far less noticeable. It does however have the advantage of speeding up your metabolism.

It is important to realize that there are situations where the two different forms of exercise tend to blur into one another. For example, if you start out walking slowly, then that is aerobic exercise, but if you start to push your speed until you reach jogging and then running pace, the expansion and contraction of your muscles means that you are also exercising anaerobically as well as aerobically.

There are a couple more factors to bear in mind.

Firstly, somewhat counter-intuitively, the heavier you are, the more calories you will burn. As you will see from the table in the next subsection, while a 120 pound person will burn fractionally over 9 cal per minute when jogging, a 180 pound person will use just short of 14 cal per minute doing exactly the same thing.

Secondly, even within a category of exercise, some forms of exercise are more effective for burning of fat than others. As an example, because of the effects of gravity, weight-bearing exercises such as jogging, running and walking are more effective for burning fat than would be non weight-bearing activities such as swimming or even cycling. In both of these cases, the effects of gravity have little or no influence on the amount of work you need to do.

No special equipment is needed, so no excuses... If you have not been doing any form of exercise recently, you should start slowly and build up gradually, but there is no reason and definitely no excuse for not starting to take exercise on a regular basis. If you're serious about losing the extra fat, half an hour or even an hour of walking every day should be a small price to pay.

You should also note that the calories burned during exercise shown in the previous table is a gross figure, and takes no account of the calories that you would have burned if you were doing something else.

For example, if you are a 180 pound person who is running and therefore burning 17 calories a minute, you would need to subtract the calories that you have been burning doing something else from this figure to arrive at any meaningful net total of extra calories burnt.

Even if the alternative activity is nothing more strenuous than sitting on the couch watching the TV, you're still burning 1.7 calories an hour according to the 'Sitting quietly' figure shown in the table. Thus, your net extra calorie burn is actually 15.3 calories a minute. I know that this might seem like a very small difference but it is important to understand that there is a difference between gross and net calories burned.

Other important exercise considerations...

One thing that is often noticeable with people who have not been exercising on a regular basis, is that they are mechanically inefficient. Even with walking, if you have not been walking in any serious way in the recent past, the chances are that your walking 'style' and pattern is likely to be inefficient at first. Injuries and other physical damage are far more likely to happen in these early days, hence not trying to do too much, too soon.

Here is the most interesting thing about being mechanically inefficient in this way. Because you are expending energy on both the exercise that you are attempting to do and on making sure you do it properly, you will in fact burn more calories in these early days than you will later once you have acquired mechanical efficiency.

To get some idea of what I mean by mechanical efficiency, think of Olympic race walkers. Could you seriously consider walking 50 km at the speed that these people go at?

An Olympic 50 km race walking champion can do it because they are mechanically efficient. Despite the fact that they probably look slightly absurd to the untrained eye, with their hips swiveling, arms pumping and walking at a speed that falls marginally short of a jog, it's amazing to think that these people really do know what they are doing.

They do, because otherwise they would not be able to walk the distances they cover at the speeds that they achieve and maintain.

Now, I'm not suggesting that you adopt the walking style of an Olympic race walker, but you should appreciate that in the early days when you first start exercising, you are mechanically awkward. Consequently, you will burn more fat calories because you are fighting your inefficiency and exercising at the same time. It follows that the more you exercise the more efficient you will become and therefore the fewer calories you will burn.

I know that sounds a little unfair, but that is just the way it is.

In a similar way, you have already seen that the bigger you are, the more calories you are going to burn. It is therefore logical that as you lose the unwanted pounds and your weight starts to fall, you will again use fewer calories while exercising than you did at the beginning.

There is nothing that you can do about this, because it is something that happens which is unavoidable.

Another aspect of adopting an exercise program for the first time is realizing that it makes a difference to your life in many ways. For example, if you spend an hour or two in the gym every day, it is logical that you will be fairly exhausted. It would be no surprise if you found that you needed an afternoon nap, something that you had previously never considered.

During the time that you are sleeping, you are burning off the minimum number of calories, so to a certain extent, this will offset the benefits of the rigorous exercise that you have just undertaken.

If you put yourself through such a strenuous, vigorous exercise regime, it will probably increase your appetite too. It is not unknown for people who decide to exercise so vigorously to put on weight rather than lose it, because they are building muscle mass at the same time as eating far more than they were previously.

Keep a journal…

As soon as you start your fat weight loss program, the first thing that you must do is start a journal.

In this journal, record all of the exercise that you do, noting the type of exercise you have been doing, how long you are doing it for and the intensity of your activity.

For example, you can walk extremely slowly or you can walk at the speed of an Olympic race walker and there is going to be a significant difference between the calories you would burn off in these two alternative scenarios, so having a record of activity intensity is essential.

Remember that when you first exercising again, you are mechanically inefficient and heavy, and that the number of calories you're burning off is therefore larger.

On the other hand, as you become more used to regular exercise, you should be able to 'up' the intensity level so that you burn off the same number of calories as you did in the early days, or perhaps even more.

Eat to Lose Weight

Don't forget to take this into account, and factor this in when you try to calculate a 'net calories burned' figure for recording in your journal.

You need to keep a constant record of your (declining) weight in this journal, plus a complete record of everything you eat and drink.

This journal will become your 'fat loss bible' over the coming weeks, and you should not underestimate the importance of keeping a journal of this nature because it can serve many positive purposes.

Firstly, there will be times when you will be tempted to skip an exercise session or tuck into a large bowl of ice cream with chocolate sauce. One quick glance at your journal should dissuade you from this (at least most of the time anyway!).

Secondly, I have no doubt that by following a regular program of exercise combined with eating and drinking in the way I recommend later in this manual, your weight will fall and you will become both slimmer and fitter.

When you are trying to lose weight, there is nothing more encouraging or inspiring than to see actual written proof that what you're trying to achieve is working, and do not forget the point I raised earlier about having a final target weight and sticking to it.

You should not realistically expect to see a massive weight loss every day unless you start off from being very obese indeed.

For this reason, I would not recommend that you take a note of your weight every day, but perhaps do so once or twice a week.

In this way, the weight loss becomes far more apparent, which is much more encouraging and far more likely to keep you going when temptation strikes from time to time (as it inevitably will).

But I don't have time for exercise...

Hogwash!

I understand that you are probably very busy every day of your life, but the fact is, everyone can make time for exercise if they apply some creative thinking and have enough determination to push through with what needs to be done.

For example, if you take the train, subway or bus to the office or factory every day, get off to three stops early and walk the rest of the way. It might add 10 minutes to your trip, but it will also provide the exercise that you must do if you are serious about shedding the fat.

In a similar way, if you use your own car to get to work, park it further away from the office if possible, and walk the rest of the way. If not, park on a lower level of the car park than you normally use, but use the stairs to get up to the floor you work on, rather than the elevator.

In fact, use the stairs whenever you can, because according to one sports nutrition expert, a person weighing 150 pounds will burn 12.5 calories per minute climbing stairs. If you work in an office block, use your break time or 15 minutes of your lunch to do some serious step climbing, and you will be making a significant impression on the 3500 calories that you have to burn to get rid of one pound of fat.

Perhaps you are a person who is extremely busy at work and equally busy at home with the family? You may even be a housewife or househusband, but there is still no excuse not to exercise.

For example, why not create a program of enjoyable exercise that the whole family can indulge in? Walking around the park, cycling or swimming together are all excellent exercise options and something that everyone can enjoy together. And, if you have children who are not yet able to swim, there is no better time to start teaching them than right now because swimming is a skill that could save their life one day.

Here's another thought.

Even everyday 'around the house' activities burn off the calories with washing the car, vacuuming the house, or digging the garden, all representing a form of activity and exercise.

So, if you usually take the car to a drive-through car wash every week, save yourself some money and get a workout every weekend by washing the car yourself.

If you vacuum the house or apartment once or twice a week, double the times that you do it. Not only will this make sure that you keep the house that much cleaner, which itself can have health benefits – cleaner air with less floating dust that can cause allergies – it will double the number of calories you burn doing basic housework as well.

If you have a garden, it could always be made to look neater and tidier couldn't it?

Once again, if you only 'do' the garden once a month, double up and double up the number of fat calories you are burning off at the same time.

Chapter 8- Get Rid of Belly Fats and the Benefits of Losing Weight

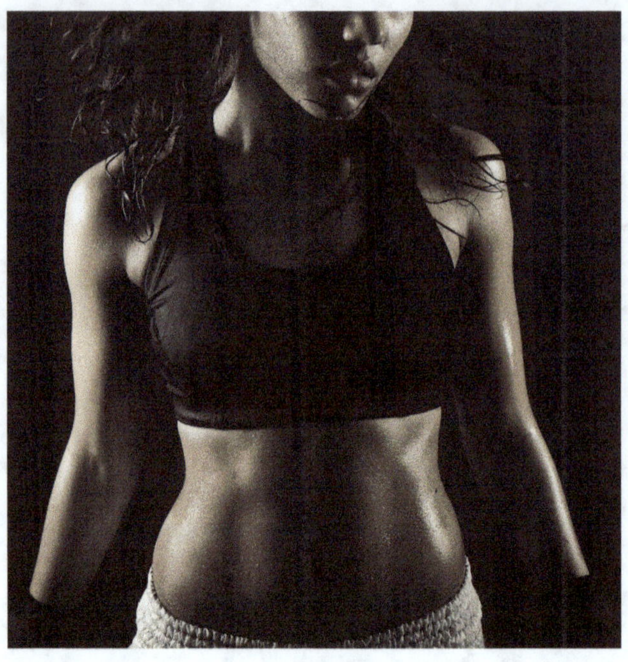

Usually, belly fat is subcutaneous fat, which is underneath the skin.

If you have problems with abdominal fat, it may also be visceral fat. This is also known as organ fat that is packed between your internal organs. This is also known as the "pot belly" or the "beer belly." It is associated with type 2 diabetes, cardiovascular disease, and colorectal cancer.

In recent studies, scientists have come to realize that it isn't really how much a person weighs—it's their amount of body fat that truly indicates obesity.

Throughout the 1980's and 90's imaging techniques were developed that helped improve the understanding of exactly how many health risks can be associated with the accumulation of body fat. These include tomography and magnetic resonance which help divide masses of tissue in the abdominal region.

For women, belly fat is more common after menopause.

Sometimes, those people who just think this goes hand-in-hand with getting older, and don't realize the danger it can cause. While women feel like it is just something that makes them go up a size in their jeans, it does carry health risks.

Like fat in any other area, it is determined by balancing your calories you take in with the energy you burn. In other words, if you eat too much and burn too little, you'll have excess fat. As you get older, your muscle mass reduces. Your fat, however, increases. When your muscle mass reduces, it also reduces the rate your body uses calories. This can make it even more difficult for people to maintain a weight that is healthy as they age.

Sometimes, you can have an increase of belly fat as you age without even gaining weight. In women, this can be due to a reduced level of estrogen. Research has shown that estrogen seems to influence where the fat is distributed in a woman's body.

Regardless of a weight shown as normal on the BMI measurement charts, women with a large waistline have been known to carry the risk of premature death and often dye earlier of cardiovascular disease.

Most women hate to even have an inch or so too much belly fat. How do you know, however, if the belly fat you carry is a health risk? Just measure it. Use a tape measure and place it around your bare stomach. You want it to be snug, but not cut into the skin. For women, if your measurement is over 35 inches, you'll be at a greater risk for health problems. For men, the measurement of concern is around 40 inches.

People who are plagued with belly fat often exercise and participate in healthy activities, yet they still retain that unwanted fat. It seems like the fat is immune to exercise. So how do you get rid of it? What is the magic combination that says "poof" to that extra poundage? It depends on your sex, age, and the amount of pounds you want to lose, but there are many tips to help you reduce that unwanted belly fat.

Benefits of Losing Weight

Losing weight isn't always easy, and as a result, it can have a negative effect on your self esteem. It is, however, important for you to main the normal weight for more than cosmetic reasons.

You need to maintain the proper health for many health reasons. In a society like ours, where people put such an importance on the way we look, feeling unattractive can lead to serious depression.

While not all overweight people get depressed, some are, in fact, quite happy the way they are, it can lead to serious emotional and mental problems in addition to the other health problems.

It can be difficult to determine how much weight you need to lose to be healthy. You should realize, however, that you don't have to lose weight if you're not actually overweight. More important than weight, is the amount of fat content you have in your body and where that fat has accumulated. Sometimes, you have weight gain because you've started working out and developed muscles.

Muscles are heavier than fat, so don't be shocked if all that exercise has reduced inches but increased weight. If this is the case, there's no problem at all and you don't have to worry about losing that weight.

While being too worried about our weight can be a problem too, knowing you're overweight and taking the steps to reduce that weight is important. There are many benefits to losing weight.

Here are a few of them:

• Reduces your risk of long-term health problems that could shorten your life. These include health problems such as diabetes and cardiovascular disease. Usually, this is the main reason people find to lose weight.

• Feeling better, healthier, and having more energy. You'll be able to take the stairs, or walk from the far end of the parking lot without losing your breath.

• Less pain in your joints. Problems such as osteoarthritis in your knees and pain and swelling in your ankles can greatly be reduced. Being overweight puts a strain on them that you will feel greatly reduced when you lose weight.

• Many times when you lose weight, especially if you're diabetic or have high blood pressure, your doctor will be able to take you off your medication. Not only will you be healthier and not taking so much medication, you'll save a lot of money at the pharmacy counter.

• You'll feel better about yourself as you gradually join the people with smaller mid sections. Your self esteem will increase. You'll find yourself interacting with others in a whole new way.

Eat to Lose Weight

• When you are eating out with co-workers you won't be overeating, so it could advance your career. Believe it or not, behavior specialists have studied this, and they found that eating healthy gives you the impression of a person that is outcome driven. This is something supervisors look for. When they see it in you, they take a closer look at you as an employee. Don't be surprised if you're looked at for a promotion you never thought you'd get.

• Save money—this is a given. If you eat less, naturally you won't be buying as much food when you eat out and when you eat at home. You'll save money all the way around. You could even put aside the extra money you normally spend on food. When your weight loss is complete, you could have enough money for a whole new wardrobe or a nice vacation to treat yourself. After all, you'll look great. You will have worked hard, so you deserve a treat.

• Keep your sex drive and be more satisfied sexually—this is especially true for men. There have been studies that show if a man is around 30 pounds overweight, he can have testosterone levels of a man that is at least 10 years older. This reduces their sex drive. Other tests have also shown that people who are obese are much less satisfied with their sexual experiences. Sex is an important part of your life, especially for those in a relationship. You want to get the most out of it. Stay fit and you will.

• You can have more friends—Face it...overweight people can sometimes be outcasts. Sometimes, it's self-inflicted, but other times, people just stay away from the "fat" person. When you lose weight, you'll feel more like making friends. You'll be able to participate in more activities which will allow you to meet more people. You'll make friends from circles you didn't dream of before.

• Influence others—sometimes, especially in spouses, one losing weight can be a positive influence on others and cause them to lose weight as well. If your children are overweight as well, it could be a genetic issue. Influencing them to begin losing weight before it gets as "out of control" as it is for you can give them a head start on the genetic problem and like Barney says, "Nip it!"

CHAPTER 9- 101 TIPS ON HOW TO LOSE WEIGHT NATURALLY

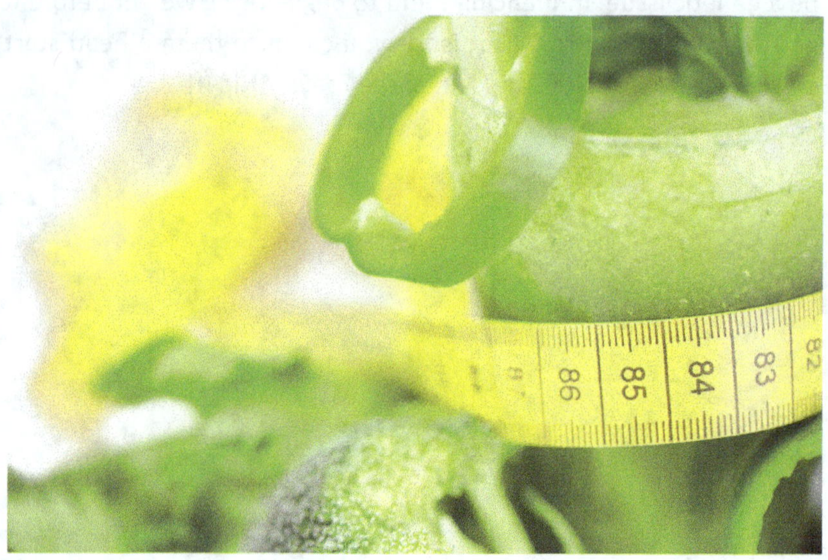

Tip # 1

Drink plenty of water. Water is not just way to flush out toxins. If you have more water in your body you will generally feel healthier and more fit. It also helps you feel full, so you don't have the urge to eat so much. And water has no calories at all.

Tip # 2

Start your day with a glass of water. It's a wonderful way to start you day. A glass of water lubricates your insides. You can still have your morning cup of tea, but have it after a glass of water.

Tip # 3

Drink a glass of water before you eat each meal. Water takes up space in your stomach, so you feel fuller without eating as much.

Tip # 4

Have another glass of water while you are having your meal. Again this is another way of making yourself full. Instead of drinking it all at once, take a sip after each bite of food. It will help the food settle and you'll feel full faster.

Tip # 5

Stay away from sweetened bottle drinks, especially sodas. They are full of sugar and calories.

Tip # 6

Include foods that contain more water, like tomatoes and watermelons. They contain 90 - 95 % water, so feast on them as much as you like. They fill you up without adding pounds.

Tip # 7

Eat fresh fruit instead of drinking fruit juice. Juice is often sweetened with sugar, but fresh fruit has natural sugars. When you eat fruit, you are taking in a lot of fiber, which the body needs, and fruit is an excellent source of vitamins.

Tip # 8

If you have a craving for fruit juice, try making your own. There are lots of juicing machines on the market.

Tip # 9

Choose fresh fruit instead of processed fruit. Processed and canned fruit does not have as much fiber as fresh fruit and processed and canned fruit is nearly always sweetened with sugar.

Tip # 10

Increase your fiber intake. Your body needs a lot of fiber, so try to include it in your diet. Eat as many fruits and vegetables as you can.

Tip # 11

Eat lots of vegetables. Leafy green vegetables are the best. Include a salad in your meal plan every day.

Tip # 12

Eat intelligently. Choose your foods wisely. Instead of grabbing chips or candy bars, grab a fruit or vegetable.

Tip # 13

Watch what you eat. Sometimes the garnishes can be richer than the food itself. Accompaniments can be very rich too.

Tip # 14

Control your sweet tooth. Sweets generally mean calories. You don't have to cut sweets out of your diet completely, but eat them in moderation. Every sweet you put in your mouth adds fat cells to your body.

Tip # 15

Develop a meal schedule and stick to it. Try to have food at fixed times of the day. You can stretch these times by half an hour, but anything more is going to affect your eating pattern.

Tip # 16

Eat only when you are hungry. Some of us have a tendency to eat whenever we see food.

Tip # 17

Quit snacking between meals. The main problem with most snacks and junk food is, they are usually less filling and contain a lot of fat and calories.

Tip # 18

Snack on vegetables if you have to snack.

Tip # 19

Go easy on tea and coffee. Tea and coffee are harmless by themselves, but when you add cream and sugar they become fattening. Having a cup of tea or coffee with cream and sugar is as bad as having a piece of chocolate cake.

Tip # 20

Drink black tea/coffee. Black tea or coffee can actually be good for you. But personally I would like to recommend tea rather than coffee. The caffeine in the coffee is not really good for you because it is an alkaloid and can affect other functions of your body like the metabolism.

Tip # 21

Count the calories as you eat. Check the label of any packaged product for the number of calories and the serving size. For unpackaged food, buy a calorie counting book.

Tip # 22

If you consume more calories than you should one day, add a bit of extra physical activity to your routine for the following day.

Tip # 23

Stay away from fried foods. The oil used for frying penetrates into the food and adds unwanted calories.

Tip # 24

Do not skip meals. The worst things you can do while watching your weight is skip a meal. It has just the opposite effect of what you want. You need to have at least three regular meals every day.

Tip # 25

Fresh vegetables are better than cooked or canned vegetables. Try to eat your vegetables raw. When you cook them, you are removing nearly half the vitamins.

Tip # 26

One egg a day. It's best if you reduce your egg intake to three a week. If you're in the habit of eating eggs every day, limit your eggs to one a day maximum.

Tip # 27

Make chocolates a luxury and not a routine.

Tip # 28

Choose a variety of foods from all food groups every day. In addition to helping you lose weight, it also helps your body fight deficiency diseases. Change the foods you eat each day so you do not get bored of your diet.

Tip # 29

Very limited or no alcoholic beverages.

Tip # 30

Try to have breakfast within one hour of waking up, so your body can charge itself with the energy it needs for the day. Breakfast is the most important meal of the day, but it does not mean that it should be the most filling meal of the day.

Tip # 31

50% - 55% of your diet should be carbohydrates. It is a myth that you should try and avoid carbohydrates when you are on a diet. Carbohydrates are an instant source of energy.

Tip # 32

25% - 30% of your diet should be proteins. Protein is an active part of keeping your body healthy.

Tip # 33

Fats should only be 15% - 20 % of your diet

Tip # 34

Try and adopt a vegetarian style diet. A vegetarian diet is healthy, but research has shown it often is missing vital minerals that come from eating meat. If you try a vegetarian diet, allow yourself to eat meat on the weekends.

Tip # 35

Choose white meat rather than red. White meat, which includes fish and fowl, is healthier than red meat.

Tip # 36

High Fiber multigrain breads are better than white breads. Multigrain breads allow you to increase your fiber and protein intake.

Tip # 37

Reduce your intake of pork. Pork is not something that can help you to lose weight. So the lesser pork you eat the better chances you have of losing weight. And remember that pork includes the pork products as well, things like bacon, ham and sausages.

Tip # 38

Limit your sugar intake. Use sugar substitutes to sweeten your food. They are just as sweetening, but not fattening.

Tip # 39

Graze 5 to 6 times a day. Instead of sticking to just three meals a day, try grazing. Grazing means having 5 or 6 smaller meals instead of three large meals. It is an excellent way of having smaller quantities of food.

Tip # 40

Eat cheat food occasionally, but only for flavor. There are many foods you need to avoid in your diet, but you may have an undying craving for them. Do not avoid them altogether. Indulge in them once in a while, but only in moderation. Don't use them to fill up, but simply to fill a craving. Enjoy the flavor.

Tip # 41

Watch your fat intake. Each fat gram contains 9 calories. By knowing the total calories and the quantity of fat in your food, you can estimate the percentage of fat. Fat content should not exceed 30%.

Tip # 42

Go easy on salt. Too much salt is one of the causes of obesity.

Tip # 43

Change from butter to cholesterol free butter. It tastes the same, but is much healthier for you.

Tip # 44

Instead of frying food, try baking it. Baking is a healthier method of preparing food because it doesn't require excessive amounts of fat or oil.

Tip # 45

Use a non stick frying pan for your cooking so you do not have to add oil.

Tip # 46

Steam your vegetables instead of cooking them. The best option is eating your vegetables fresh, however, if you do not like eating fresh vegetables, try steaming them without adding any additional salt or seasoning. This is the healthiest way to eat cabbages, cauliflowers and a host of other vegetables.

Tip # 47

Carry parsley with you. Parsley is an excellent thing to munch on between meals. It's vitamin rich and keeps your breath fresh.

Tip # 48

Choose low fat or no fat substitutes. Although fat gives us nutrients, it also packs on the calories. It's much better to get your nutrients from proteins and carbohydrates. It's healthier for your heart too.

Tip # 49

Avoid crash diets. They are bad for your health and you will gain your weight back as soon as you stop them. Crash diets are not a solution to weight loss. You might lose a few pounds quickly, but the moment you give up on the crash diet, all your weight comes back.

Tip # 50

Develop a habit of chewing all your food including liquid food and soft foods like sweets, and ice cream, at least 8 to 12 times. This is essential to add saliva to the food, as it starts the digestion process.

Tip # 51

Dry wine is better than sweet wine. Sweet wines naturally contain a lot of sugar, but in dry wines, most of the sugar has been fermented away.

Tip # 52

When you decide it's time to start working out, start slowly and don't get discouraged if you don't achieve your fitness goals after the first week. If you try to push your body too much in the first few weeks, you are likely to end up with injuries.

Tip # 53

Check your weight before you start a training routine and keep checking for changes, but do not expect a radical drop immediately. It might be a couple weeks before you notice some change. However it is crucial that you continue to monitor your weight. As you're losing fat weight, you're gaining muscle mass, so your overall weight may not change as dramatically as you would like it to. Your size, however, will decrease, so measure your body regularly too.

Tip # 54

When you notice a change, reward yourself...but not with food. Go to a movie or buy yourself something like a new dress or accessories. This can help keep you motivated.

Tip # 55

Take a day off from exercise every week. Your body needs a day or two each week to relax and rejuvenate itself.

Tip # 56

Exercise outdoors as much as possible. It gives your body a chance to get fresh air and sunshine. It also keeps you perked up and it's a break from being inside all day.

Tip # 57

Exercise at home. You don't need to join a gym to exercise. You don't even need to buy exercise equipment. Visit the library or look online for exercises you can do without equipment. If you do want to get some equipment, a Wii Fit is a great investment and it makes exercising a lot of fun.

Tip # 58

Exercise with a friend. Ideally, it should be somebody committed to exercising like you or your interest might fade.

Tip # 59

Stop when your body has had enough. There is no need to push it. When you have worked out for a considerable time, your body will start giving you signals.

Listen to your body, especially in the initial stages. Take one step at a time. Stop when you are out of breath or when a certain part of your body tells you that it has had enough.

Tip # 60

Increase your exercise time gradually. Dramatic jumps in exercise time can leave your body exhausted and more prone to injury. Instead of increasing your workout routine by 30 minutes, increase it by 10 minutes a week for 3 weeks.

Tip # 61

Select an exercise pattern to suit your lifestyle. All of us have different lifestyles and professions so follow an exercise routine that is suitable for you.

Tip # 62

Don't stand, walk. If you can walk about then do so. Do not stand in a fixed position. Pacing about is a good thing to do. If you are thinking deeply about something, try pacing, it will aid in your thinking too.

Tip # 63

Don't sit, stand. If you can stand, then do not sit. The golden rule is to choose a position that is less comfortable.

Tip # 64

Don't lie down, sit. The rule that we mentioned above rings true here as well.

Tip # 65

Replace the comfortable couch and chairs in front of the TV. If you have less comfortable furniture in front of the TV, you are less likely to sit in front of it.

Tip # 66

If you have a sitting job, stand up and stretch every half hour. Most jobs today are sitting jobs that are sedentary. By stretching every half hour you help your body stay awake and your metabolism running, which helps burn fat.

Tip # 67

While making telephone calls try walking around.

Tip # 68

Use the stairs instead of the elevator whenever you can. If you have to travel to the 40th floor, take the elevator part way and walk the rest of the way.

Tip # 69

Smoking is bad for weight loss. Smoking may not contribute to weight loss but smoking leads to other conditions like erratic eating habits and excessive dependence on things like coffee.

Tip # 70

If you hate running, remember, you do not have to run a marathon to stay fit. 10 minutes of cardio each day is good enough for most people.

Tip # 71

If you can't run, try walking. 15 minutes of brisk walking a day is enough to keep most people fit.

Tip # 72

Any distance is walk able if you have the time, so consider walking to places that you would normally drive, such as work or the market if they're not too far away. It may take you longer, but the health benefits will last you a lifetime.

Tip # 73

It sounds strange, but some people have reported that they lost more weight when they drank black coffee before a workout. While there's no hard data to support this, nutritionists speculate that the caffeine in coffee makes the body rely more on fat for fuel during the work out. It's worth trying.

Tip # 74

Avoid drinking coffee in excess, as it tends to desensitize your body to the fat burning effects of caffeine.

Tip # 75

Stop using remote controls. Get up from the couch and change the TV channel manually.

Tip # 76

Often when we come home tired from work, we tend to get others to do simple chores for us. These things are no big deal. They are things that we can do for ourselves, but we don't.

Tip # 77

Walk up and down escalators as if they were normal stairs.

Tip # 78

During TV commercial breaks, get up and walk around. Reach over and touch your toes or do any simple exercise that will get the blood flowing.

Tip # 79

Wriggle your toes and your fingers whenever you can. This is a stress reliever and it gives you a chance to work your hand and leg joints.

Tip # 80

Turn on music and dance like wild. Let your hair down once in a while. Think back to the days of your wild child hood. Close the door of your room, turn on your sound system to the highest volume possible and do the wackiest dance you can think of. Jump on your bed and jump off it again. Roll all over the floor. Have fun.

Tip # 81

Carry a soft flying disc or Frisbee with you. Toss it around and get up and go get it. This is also an excellent way to beat stress. It makes you feel good to throw something. Although it's not the throwing part that you are interested in, it is the fetching part. Each time you get up to fetch, you are giving yourself a chance to stretch your muscles and joints and get your metabolism working harder to burn more fat.

Tip # 82

Park at least a block away from your destination and walk the rest of the way. You might not have time to fit long walks into your busy schedule, so this is a way to ensure you get to walk for a little bit every day. If you take the bus or the subway, get off at an earlier station and walk the rest of the way.

Tip # 83

When nobody is watching try doing pelvic gyrations. Your mid section gets the least bit of exercise so excess weight tends to settle there.

Stomach crunches might be too strenuous an exercise to start off with, but gyrations are relatively mild. Pelvic gyrations make you thrust your midsection towards all directions and this is the best way of tightening every muscle in that area.

Tip # 84

Tuck in your tummy whenever you walk. Get that proper gait and exercise your muscles at the same time.

Tip # 85

Try breathing exercises. Breathing exercises can lead to weight loss. If you are doing the breathing exercises properly, you will find that you can exert a lot of pressure on the muscles around the mid section.

You can feel a tightening of these muscles each time you breathe in or breathe out. So breathe properly, it is good for you.

Tip # 86

Try yoga. Yoga is one of the best ways of losing weight. One of the benefits of yoga is, you learn to control virtually every muscle and joint of your body so the issue of weight gain will cease to exist.

Tip # 87

Try massaging your partner. This is a fun way to lose weight. It is something that can give your partner a lot of pleasure and at the same time can help you exercise.

Tip # 88

Punch the air 50 times. It helps your cardiovascular system and jump starts your metabolism.

Tip # 89

Instead of walking up and down the stairs one at a time, take them two at a time.

Tip # 90

If you have a dog, take it for a run and let the dog lead you on. You will be surprised how much exercise a dog can give you.

Animals are sensible enough to know that they need a lot of exercise, so let your animal walk you and before you know it you'll be running.

Tip # 91

Join a dance class. Dancing is a wonderful way to burn off extra calories. When you dance, you are burning a lot of calories.

Tip # 92

Lean against a wall with your hands flat against the wall and your face very close to the wall. Use your hands to push your body away from the wall. It resembles a standing push up and is easier than lying on the floor.

Tip # 93

If there is a pool nearby, go for a swim as often as you can. Swimming is one of the best exercises to move your whole body.

Tip # 94

Play table tennis or basket ball. Games are a fun way to lose weight. It is much more exciting to play a game than just work out by yourself. The best thing about games is, they are addictive. It is something you can look forward to and there is no stress involved in the program. In fact the more you play the less you will consider this to be a part of your weight loss program. As you burn away those calories, you will also be able to expand your social circle.

Tip # 95

Any work out should start with a 5 to 10 minute warm up and should end with a 5 to 10 minute cool down session. Your body needs to reach a certain level of readiness before it can actually start responding to exercise.

Tip # 96

Do not carry your mobile phone, but leave it someplace where you can hear it ringing. When it rings, you have to get up to answer it.

Tip # 97

While traveling in an elevator, raise up on your toes and then back onto your feet again. Do this several times. Also try flexing your buttock muscles.

In fact there are many muscles in our body that we can twitch and flex without inviting the attention of others. Even if others do notice you, it's no big deal.

Tip # 98

Undress and stare at yourself in front of your mirror. If what you see displeases you, then you have more reason to work out.

Turn to your side and get a very good view of your side profile. This is an excellent way of checking whether you have a tummy that is starting to bulge or has bulged already.

Tip # 99

If you have a banister rail or a balustrade that will support you, sit on it and pump your legs as if you are riding a bicycle, taking care not to fall off. This might sound like a crazy idea, but it's fun. And fun will keep you active.

Tip # 100

Do not slouch in your chair. Maintain an erect posture with your tummy tucked in. Slouching is a very bad habit. Not only is it bad for your back, but it also gives you a very flabby figure.

Tip # 101

Breathe in as strongly as you can and tuck in your tummy as much as you can. Hold it for a few seconds and slowly release your breath, taking care not to let out your tummy. Try to keep breathing like this at least fifty or sixty times a day.

After the first day, you should feel the muscles of your stomach tightening each time you do this. Practice this for 20 days. At the end of the twentieth day, you will have lost at least an inch.

ABOUT THE AUTHOR

Judy Martin is a mother of three. Just like any other mother, she was having trouble getting back in shape. When her third child, Luke was born, she loses hope. But then she realized that she needs to stay fit and healthy. She's doing this for her children and more importantly for herself.

Judy is now a health buff and a nutritionist. She compiled everything that she learned about getting fit and put it in a book so she may be able to inspire others.